# MY SENSES
## ARE LIKE CUPS

# MY
# SENSES
# ARE LIKE CUPS

## WHAT TO DO WHEN EVERYTHING FEELS
## TOO MUCH OR NOT NEARLY ENOUGH

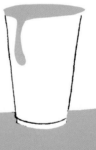

## CLARE WARD AND
## JAMIE GALPIN
### WITH JUDY COURTNEY, OT

Illustrated by Clare Ward

**Jessica Kingsley Publishers**
London and Philadelphia

# Contents

## Part 2: Small Cups, Big Cups, Medium Cups

# Foreword

I have sensory issues which can make me really, really stressed and I can get fizzy when there's shouting or annoying noises, when I have to do PE or go into the playground, when it's raining or when I'm asked to stop reading by my parents.

Before I read this book I found it hard to understand what all this means and why I sometimes feel different to lots of my friends. I really liked how the book helped me to understand my senses and what I need to help my senses calm down. I also thought that it was very calming and gentle. It made me feel like my senses are not a problem, even though they're all muddled up. It made me feel better about having sensory issues and less worried.

Emmeline Dent (age 8)

# A Note from the Authors

Hello! Thank you for looking at our book. You might be reading it because you want to find out how to feel 'just right'. Or maybe someone gave it to you.

However you got here, welcome to this book about the senses. It's about everybody's senses, especially yours, and how these senses can make us feel.

Have you ever asked yourself:

* Why do we really hate some foods?

* Why do some of us need to have music on while we do homework?

* How come it is easier for some of us to learn if we move around in lessons?

* Why do some of us prefer to wear tight clothes and some of us love looser clothes?

* How come some of us need to fidget more than others?

* Why do we sometimes have really **big** feelings that seem to come from nowhere?

If you want to find out, then this book will help. It can help us to answer all of these questions or maybe just make us more curious about what we feel and why.

This book can help in three different ways:

**1.** It can be confusing (and sometimes really annoying) to feel fidgety, overwhelmed or just 'not quite right'.

The next few pages are our way of explaining why this might happen.

**2.** It can be hard to explain to other people what's going on when we feel like this.

You can lend this book to other people to help you explain how you feel.

**3.** It can be difficult to know how to get back to feeling 'just right'.

There are some ideas at the end of this book and more online.

Oh, and one more thing! You might not know what certain words mean — **yet**. Some trickier words or phrases have ? next to them followed by a **definition**? of the word. For example:

**Definition**? = the meaning of a word or sentence.

Now you are ready to start learning about sense cups. We hope this helps.

*Clare and Jamie*

Whenever we suggest finding something online, you will find that information on this webpage: www.jkp.com/catalogue/book/9781839978470. On it, you will find examples of games and activities designed to help you get back to feeling 'just right'. There are lots of ideas to try out at home and at school, so have a look! Extra copies of all activities marked with ⬇ can be downloaded from here too.

# PART 1

# Our SENSES

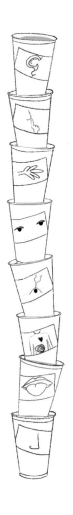

Humans have eight different senses. We use them to understand ourselves and the world around us. Some of them will be familiar to you and some might be new. We will explain more about those later on.

These are the word labels we have given our senses:

taste

touch

smell

sight

hearing

balance (vestibular [ves-tib-yu-lar])

proprioception [pro-pree-o-sep-shon]

interoception [in-ter-o-sep-shun]

Some of us might use some senses more than others. For example, if we are Deaf, we might not use our hearing sense in the same way as people who are not. If we are Deaf, we might use our sight and touch senses much more.

We are all different in how our senses work, and everyone being different is kind of what makes us all the same!

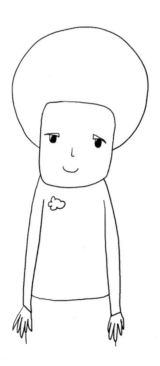

We can think about our different senses as being like cups inside us.

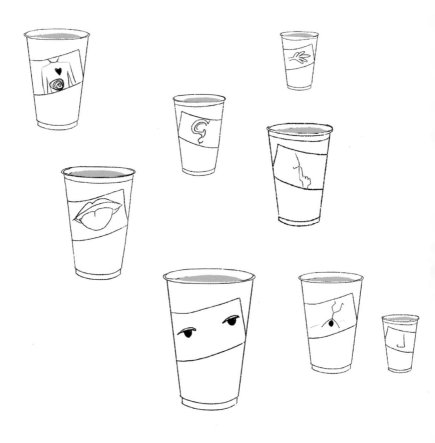

Imagine that each of our eight senses has a different cup. And when that sense cup is just about full, we get a feeling of things being 'just right'.

Information that our eight senses notice, both inside us and outside of us, is like water that can fill the eight sense cups.

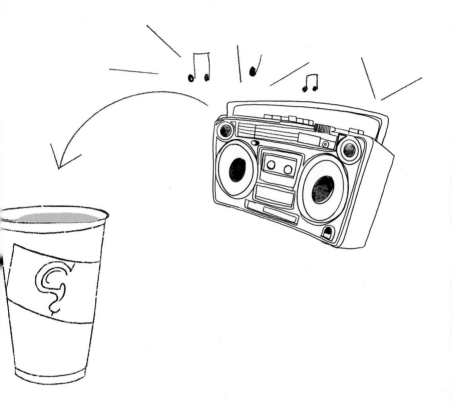

When one of our sense cups is nearly filled up, we usually have a calm and 'just right' feeling.

This book is about what might happen when we have too much or too little input or information (like water) in our sense cups.

When our senses feel too much for us:

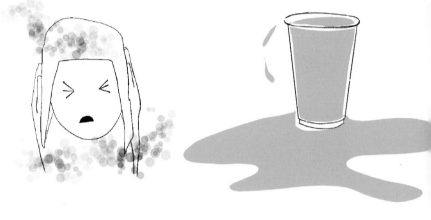

Or too little:

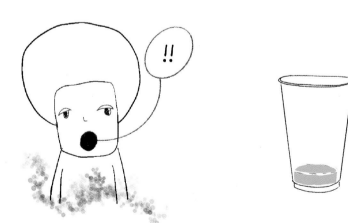

In this book, we are going to look at each sense in turn. We will help you work out if and when any of your sense cups might be overflowing or empty. **What feels 'just right' is different for each of us.**

After each sense there is a space for you to fill in to help you remember what you found out about yourself and each of your eight sense cups. The space will look like this:

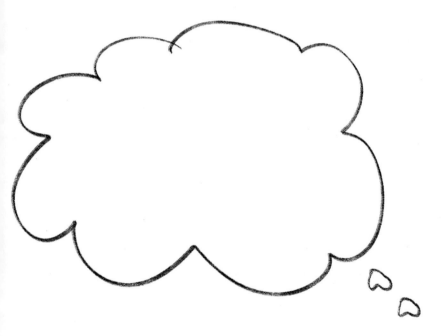

Learning about our sense cups can help us find ways to keep them at the 'just right' level that helps us feel good.

We are all very different.

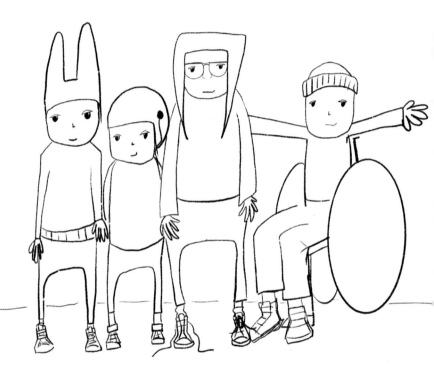

Both on the outside...

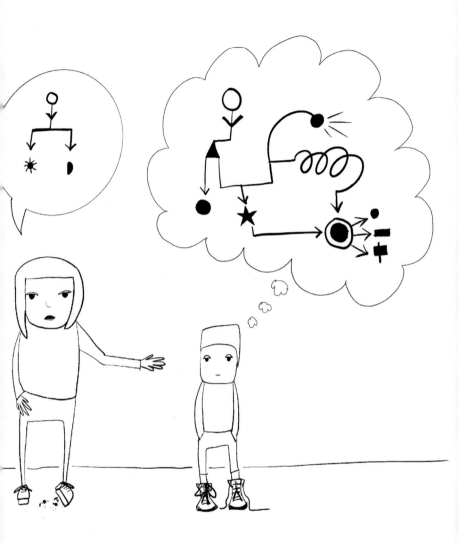

...and on the inside.

We all have differences but we also have things that make us all the same! You could even say that being different is something we all have in common!

We are all living creatures who need energy to keep going.

We try to use our energy as carefully as we can.

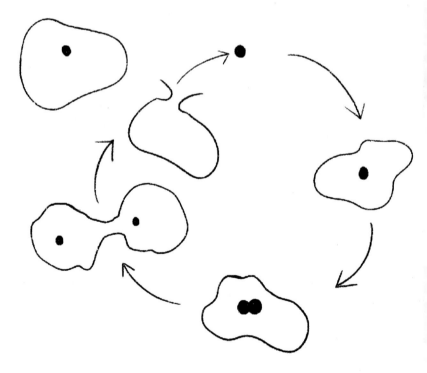

Whether we are tiny cells...

...or something bigger.

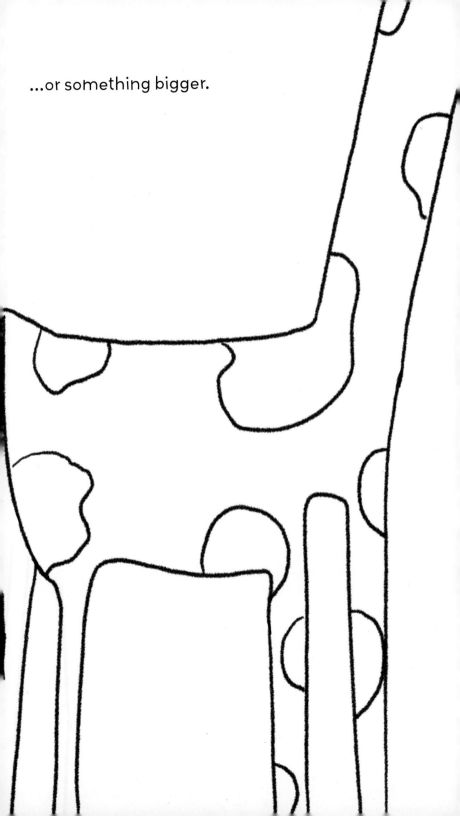

We use a lot of energy trying to understand the world around us – thinking, planning and organising. To save energy we save lots of ideas, plans and thoughts in our brains.

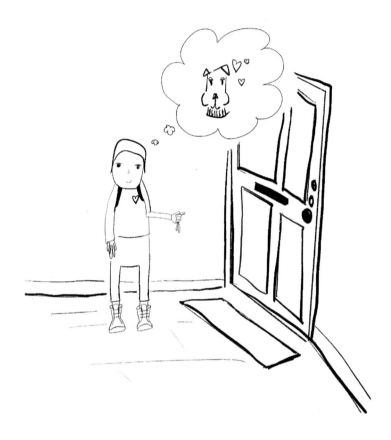

We can use these ideas, plans and thoughts to make it easier to understand the world around us. And we can use our saved ideas, plans and thoughts to make guesses about the world. These are called predictions.

Predicting things means we have an idea
of what might happen before it happens.
And then we might not have to use as much
energy to understand the world.

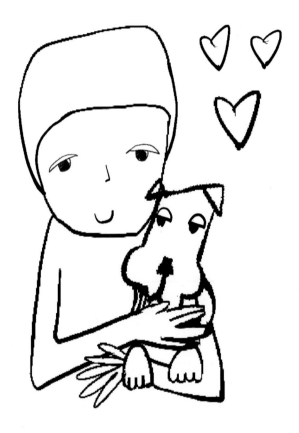

Also, when our predictions come true, we feel
happy and relaxed.

But when something unexpected happens, something we did not predict...

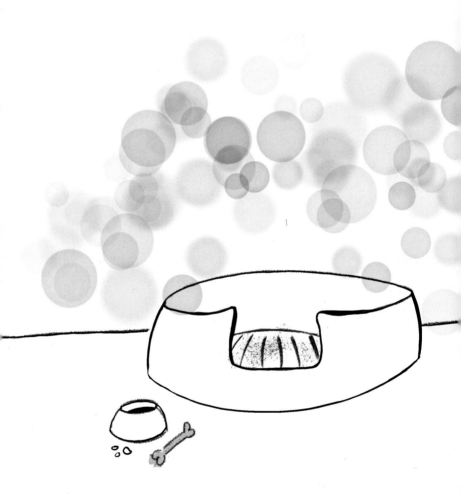

...it can make us feel stressed.

This is because it can make us feel **uncertain**?. Humans don't really like uncertainty. It can feel 'not right'.

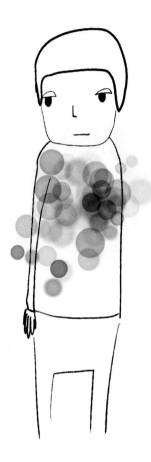

**Uncertain**? = not sure. How we might feel when we don't know what's going to happen.

We can feel uncertain for lots of different reasons.

We might feel uncertain when we meet someone new. We call this social uncertainty.

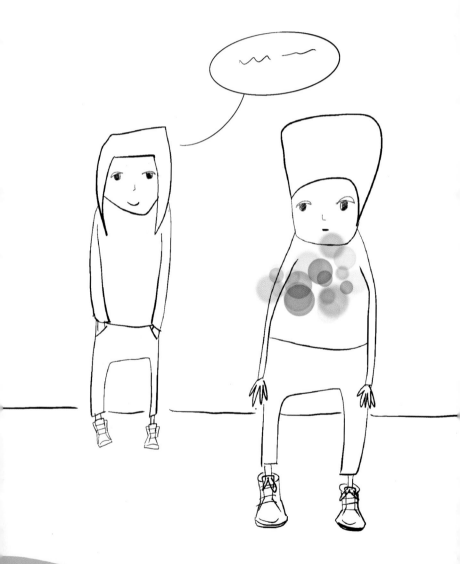

We might feel uncertain when our timetable is changed. We call this structural uncertainty.

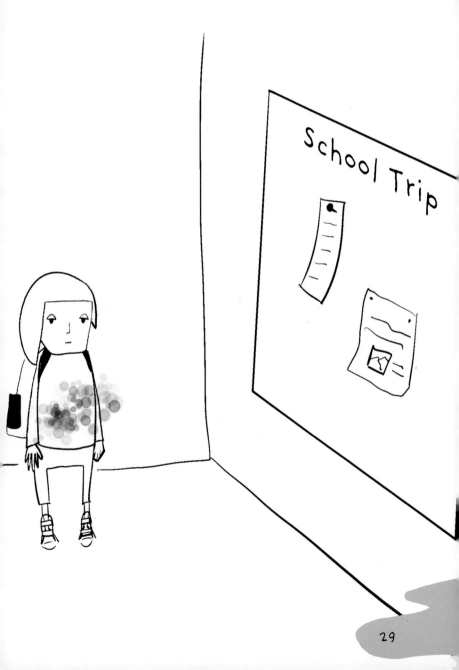

We might get sensory uncertainty too...

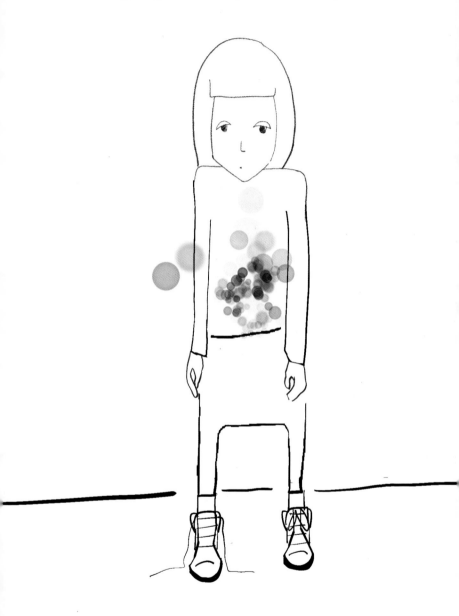

...and that's what this book is about.

Different parts of our body collect sensory information about what's around us (what we are experiencing) and what's inside us (how we are feeling, are we hungry, tired, thirsty?).

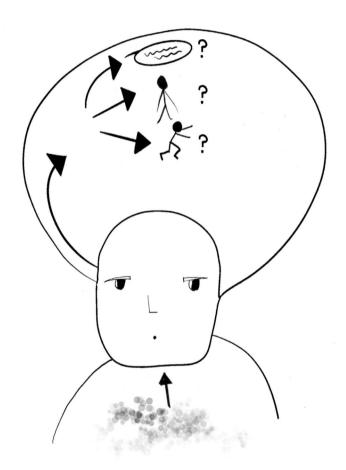

The parts of our body send the sensory information to our brain where we work out what to do about it.

It's a very clever system.

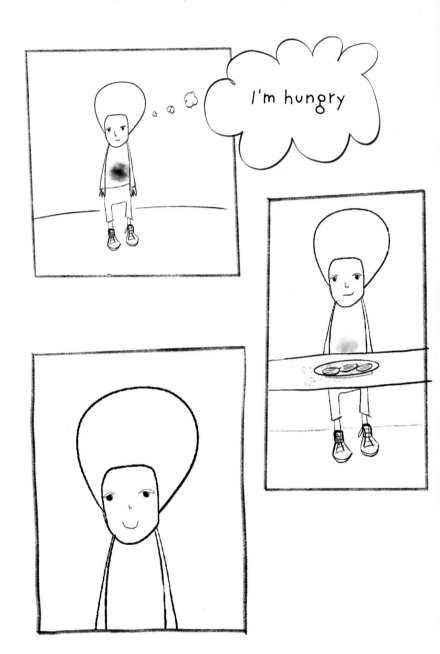

Sometimes this system does not help us as much as it could.

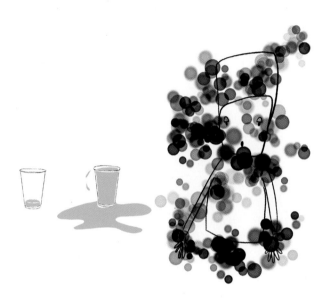

When we get too much sensory information from one of our senses, or not enough, it could make us feel all bouncy, sad, angry or just 'not right'.

Things will feel uncertain. It's our body's way of telling us that we need to do something to get back to feeling 'just right'.

We are going to look at each of our sense cups and what it might be like if they get too empty or start to overflow.

Let's look more closely at our senses and how we use them to understand the world. For each sense you will find examples of things that might be signs that a sense cup is too full or too empty. At the end of the book and online, there are some ideas for what to do to get back to feeling 'just right'. We hope you enjoy experimenting with them!

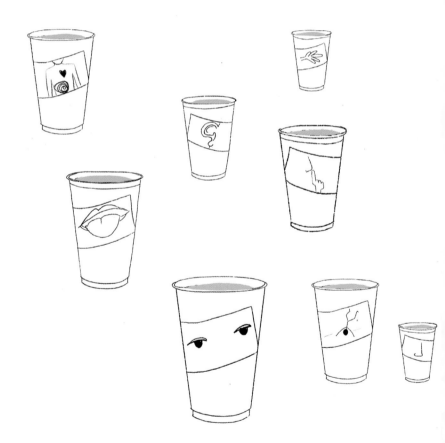

We have lots of different senses. Can you remember how many we said at the start of the book? That's right. Eight.

Do you remember what they all are?

taste                    touch

smell                    sight

hearing                  balance
                         [ves-tib-yu-lar]

proprioception
[pro-pree-o-sep-          interoception [in-
shon]                    ter-o-sep-shun]

You probably know more about taste, touch, smell, sight and hearing. They are the ones we talk about the most.

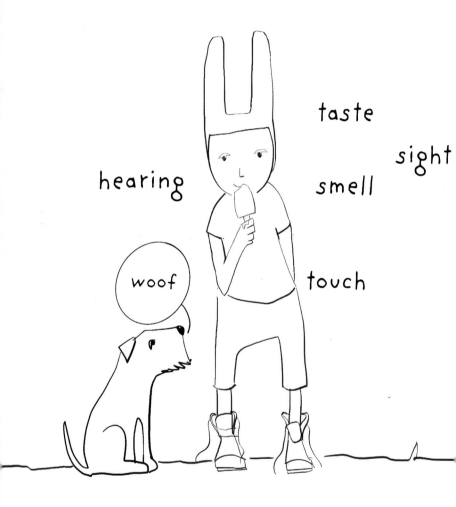

taste

sight

hearing

smell

woof

touch

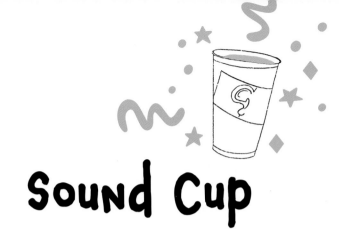

# Sound Cup

Sometimes our sound cup gets too full (with too much noise or sounds that are confusing)...

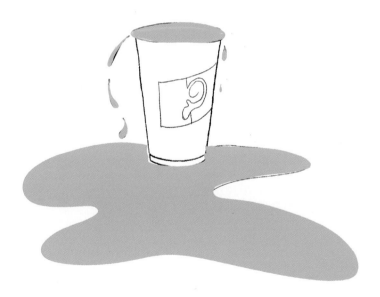

...and we need to do things to empty it.

Some of us might need to...

* listen to our favourite music
(on headphones or out loud)

* put our hands over our ears

* make our own sounds (humming,
whistling, singing or talking)

* stay away from loud places
(like playgrounds or school canteens)

* avoid unpredictable noises
(like balloons or funfairs).

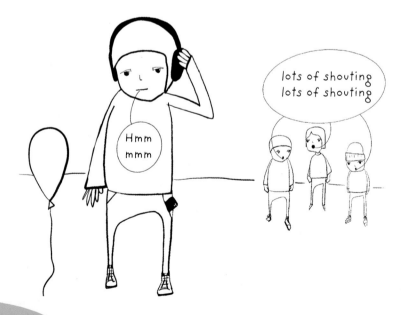

Other times our sound cup might be empty
and need filling up...

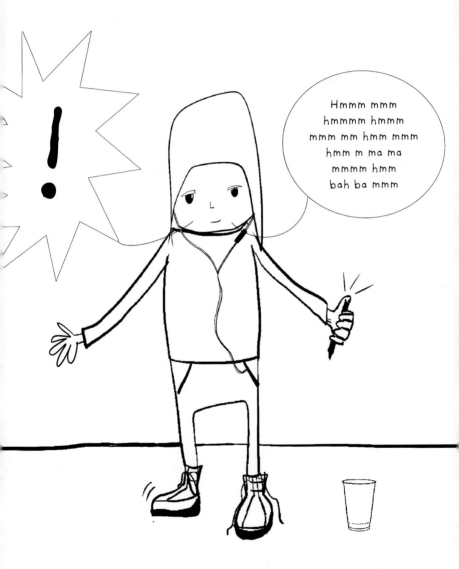

...so we can get back to the calm, 'just right'
feeling.

Some of us might need to...

☐ listen to music (on headphones or out loud) lots of the time

☐ make our own sounds (humming, whistling, beatboxing, singing, talking to ourselves, drumming, tapping or shaking things)

☐ shout out

☐ do our homework in a noisy room

☐ play loud games

☐ fidget with things that make a sound.

Tick anything that you do. Write in the bubble anything else you might feel the need to do when your sound cup overflows (too much noise!) or needs filling up (it's too quiet!).

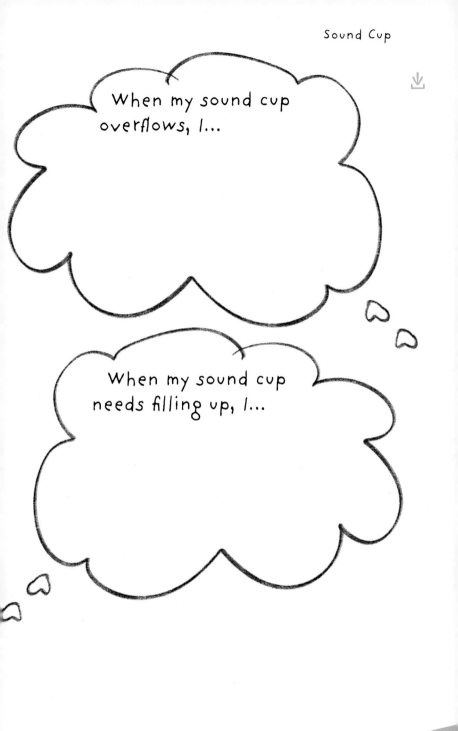

Remember! At the end of the book and online, there are some more ideas for what to do to get back to feeling 'just right'.

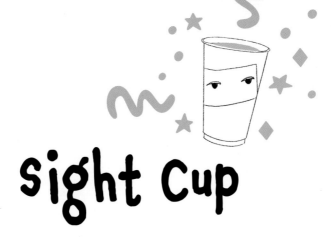

# Sight Cup

If our sight cup is full of information that we find 'too much' or we can't make sense of, we might feel the need to do things like...

* keep lighting low

* work in a clear space, without too many pictures or colours

* put things in order and tidy up

* wear plain clothes that don't have a pattern

* keep things neat in rows or symmetrical

...to cut down the amount of stuff we are seeing (some people call this 'visual noise').

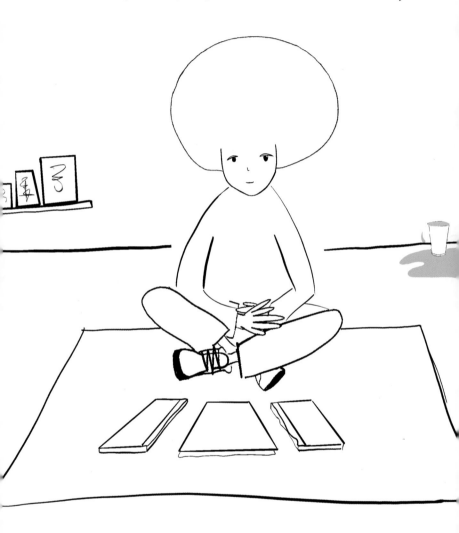

Sometimes our sight cup has not got enough in it and we need to do things like...

* work in a space with lots of colour and objects in it

* decorate everything

* wear bright or patterned clothes

* be a bit messy

...to fill it up and get back to a calmer, 'just right' feeling.

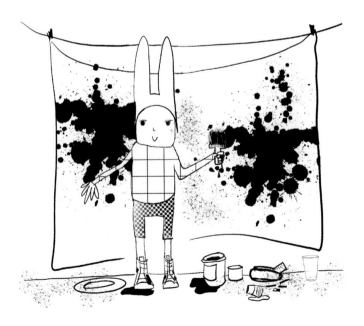

## What about **you**?

Do you feel better when your bedroom is:

☐ tidy      ☐ clean

☐ messy      ☐ don't mind?

Tick whichever options feel like you most of the time. Write in the bubble what kind of space you learn and work best in.

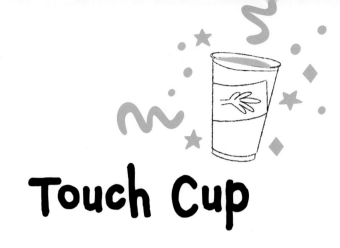

# Touch Cup

If our touch cup is full of information about textures we don't like or find overwhelming, we do whatever we can to empty it.

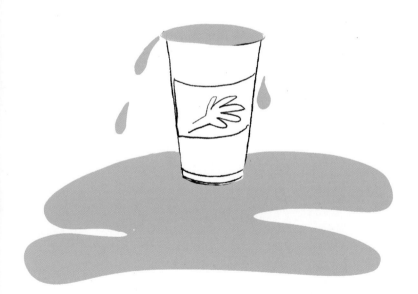

We might feel the need to do some things so we can feel 'right' again.

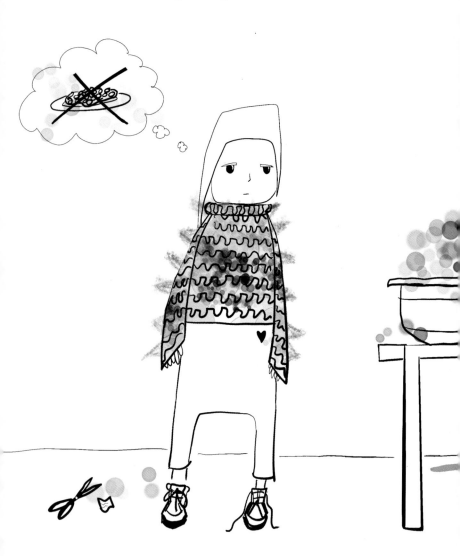

To empty our touch cup, some of us might:

- ☐ avoid certain foods we don't like the feel of

- ☐ prefer not to wear particular clothes

- ☐ say no to messy activities

- ☐ wear our sleeves over our hands

- ☐ wear our socks on the beach

- ☐ insist on always wearing our favourite clothes

- ☐ try and avoid people touching us unexpectedly

- ☐ wear clothes without labels.

Remember to tick any of these that you do too! Is there anything else that you do when your touch cup is too full?

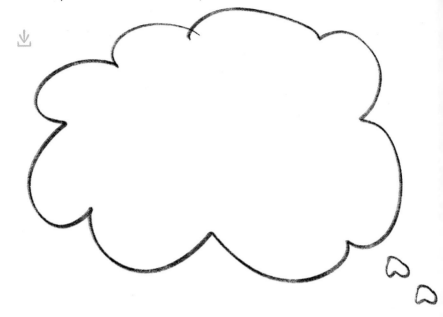

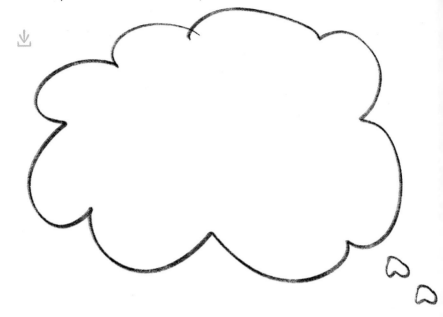

Or maybe your touch cup is almost empty and you have to do things to try and fill it up.

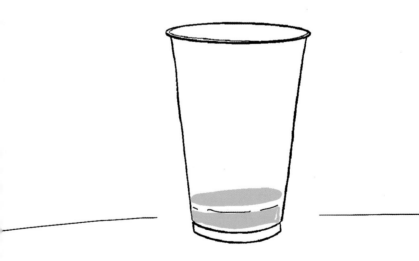

We might feel the need to move and **fidget**? ...

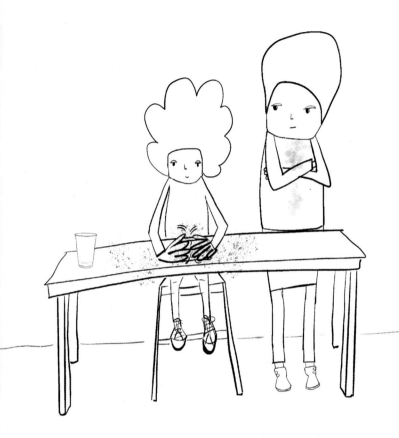

...to get back to the calm, 'just right' feeling.

**Fidgeting**? = when we move a part of our body or play with something repetitively.

Fidgeting is important. Like lots of the things we do, it is about more than one cup. At the end of the book there are some ideas on **how** to fidget so that we don't annoy people!

How do you fidget?

Write some of the things you do in the thought bubble.

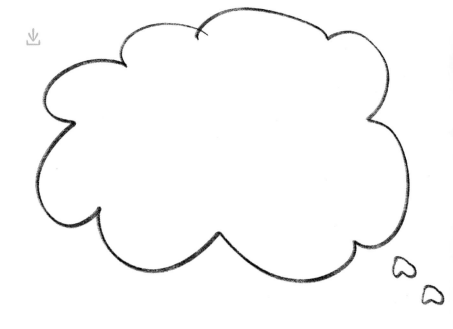

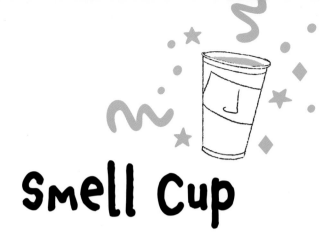

# Smell Cup

Our smell cup can also be too empty, or it can overflow with smells that we don't like or weren't expecting.

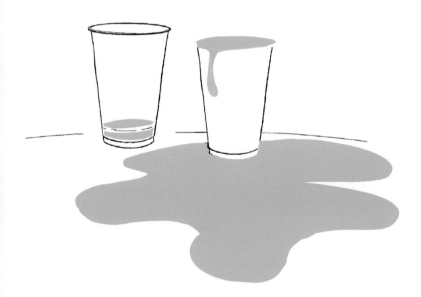

Then we have to do things to get it back to the right level.

We might feel the need to...

☐ smell familiar things

☐ avoid places with strong smells

☐ avoid people with strong perfume

☐ try to stop our favourite clothes or toys from being washed

...to get back to the calm, 'just right' feeling. Tick any of them that you do too.

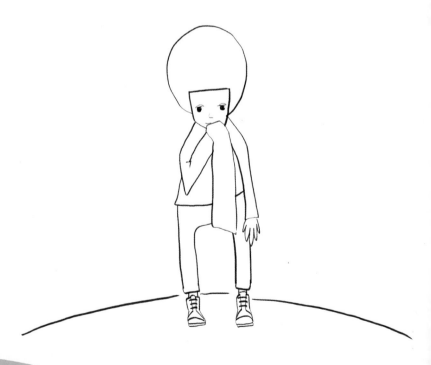

Draw or write any smells that are 'too disgusting' or 'too much' for you in the bubble.

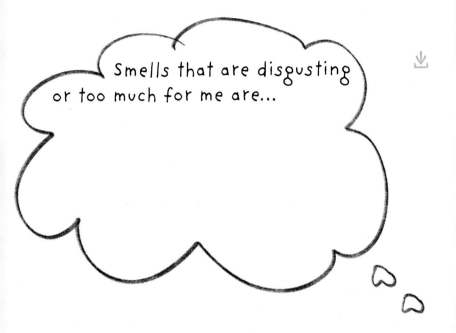

Smells that are disgusting or too much for me are...

How about good smells? Do you have any favourite smells? Write them down in the bubble.

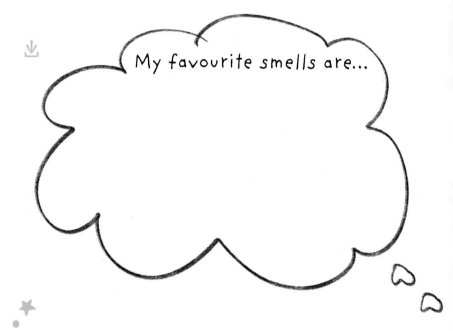

My favourite smells are...

Remember! At the end of the book and online, there are some ideas for what to do to get back to feeling 'just right' when your smell cup is empty or overflowing.

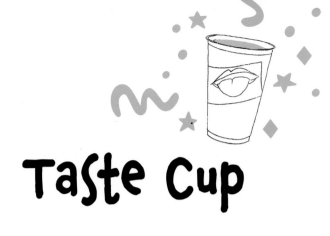

# Taste Cup

If our taste cup overflows with information that we don't like, or isn't always the same, we might feel the need to make sure this doesn't happen often.

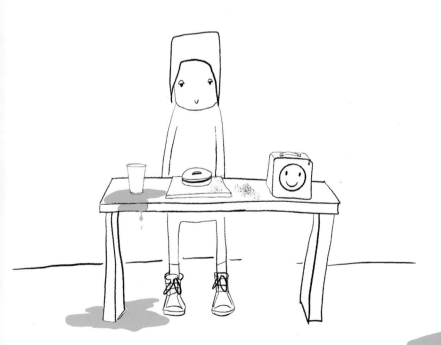

We might feel the need to...

☐ eat the same things every day

☐ eat small amounts

☐ eat things that taste the same each time

☐ eat one type of food at a time

☐ prefer plain or sweet foods

☐ always choose the same brand of our favourite foods

☐ make sure different foods don't touch.

Tick any of these that you do too.

Anything else?

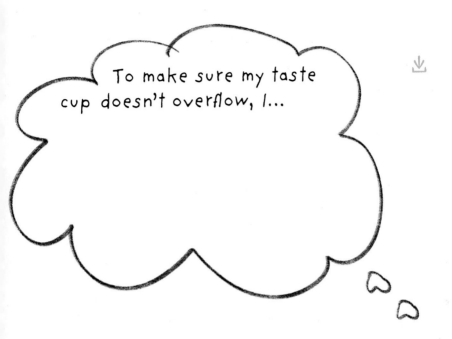

To make sure my taste cup doesn't overflow, I...

Some of us find it hard to fill up our taste cup. We need to do things to get more information in there.

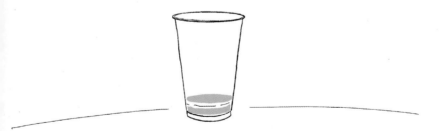

59

We might feel the need to...

☐ snack often

☐ chew stuff – not just foods

☐ eat strong tasting or spicy food

...to get back to the calm 'just right' feeling. Tick the ones you do to get back to that 'just right' feeling.

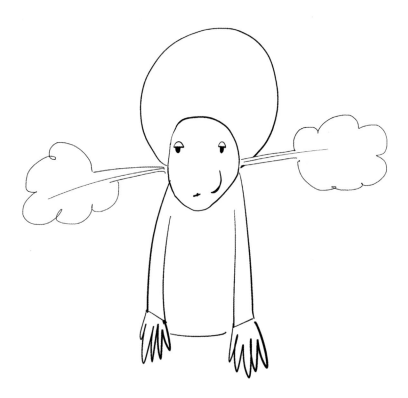

We have learnt a lot about the five senses we have just looked at. It can seem like those are the only ones we need to think about. But as we said right at the start, we have eight senses that help us understand our world. That means we have three more cups to learn about. Let's get investigating!

# Balance Cup

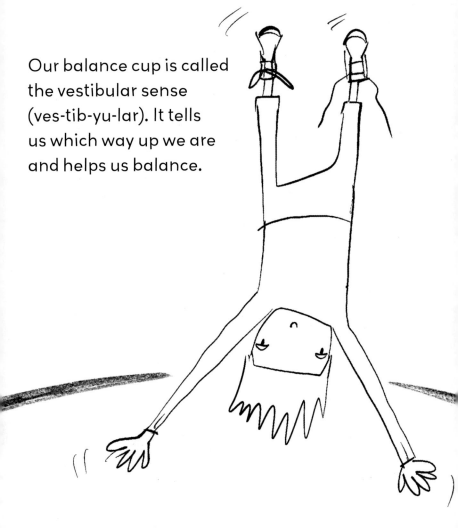

Our balance cup is called the vestibular sense (ves-tib-yu-lar). It tells us which way up we are and helps us balance.

This is why we like to call it our balance sense (and it is easier to say than vestibu? ...vesti? ...vestibular!).

Activity! Close your eyes and touch your toes a few times. How do you know when you're upright?

Now that you understand what this sense does, let's think about our balance cup.

If our balance cup doesn't have enough information in it, we might feel the need to...

☐ climb high things

☐ hang upside down

☐ spin

☐ jump around

☐ swing on a tyre swing

☐ rock in a chair

☐ hang off the back of the sofa

☐ bounce on beds

☐ go to the swings

☐ get up and down from our chair a lot

...to get back to feeling 'just right'.

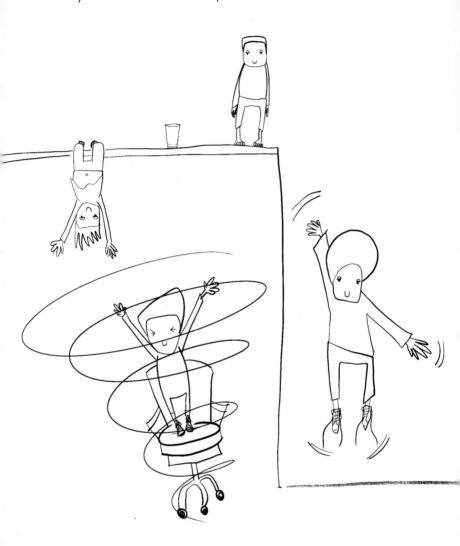

How about you? Tick the things you do in the list. Or if you do other things in lessons or at home, write them down in the bubble.

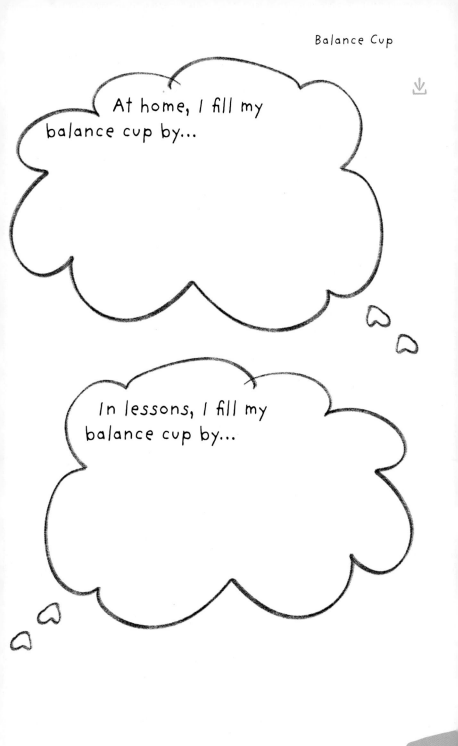

At home, I fill my balance cup by...

In lessons, I fill my balance cup by...

If our balance cup is overflowing and has too much information in it, or information that's confusing, we may feel the need to **ground ourselves**? to feel safe.

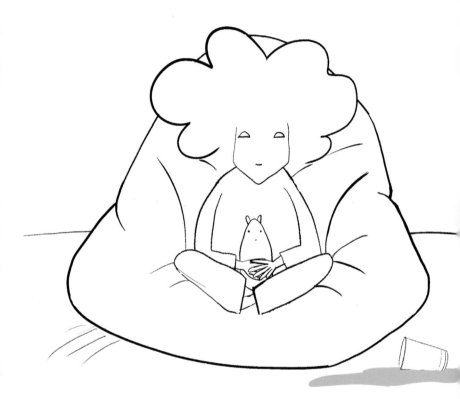

**Grounding ourselves**? = things that help us calm down and focus on what is happening **right now**.

This can be things like:

☐ being still

☐ breathing slowly

☐ noticing how different parts of our body feel.

How about you? Tick any of these things that you do.

Do you ever get a bit dizzy or feel like the world is spinning? What do you do when this happens?

Draw or write about it in the bubble.

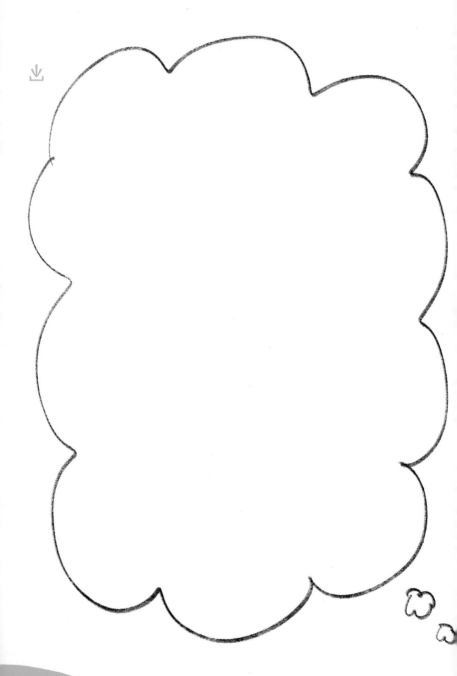

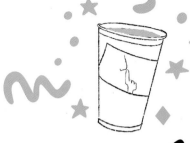

# Body Awareness Cup

The body awareness sense tells us where the different bits of us are in space. No, not intergalactic space! It tells you where you are in the room or where your legs are compared to where an object like a table or a step is.

This sense is called our proprioceptive (pro-pree-o-sep-tiv) sense, but we prefer 'body awareness' because it is easier to say!

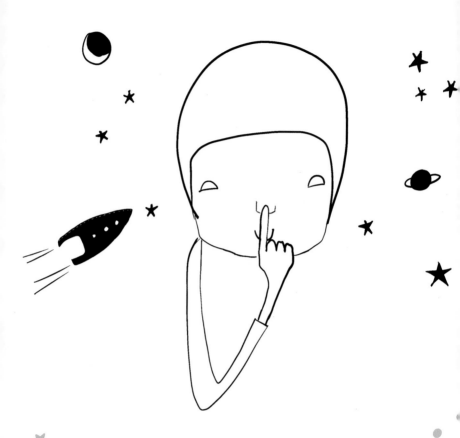

Activity! Close your eyes and see if you can touch your nose. How do you know where your nose is on your face?

We've learnt about our body awareness sense, let's now think about our body awareness cup.

If our body awareness cup is overflowing, we might feel the need to do some things to try and stay calm and happy.

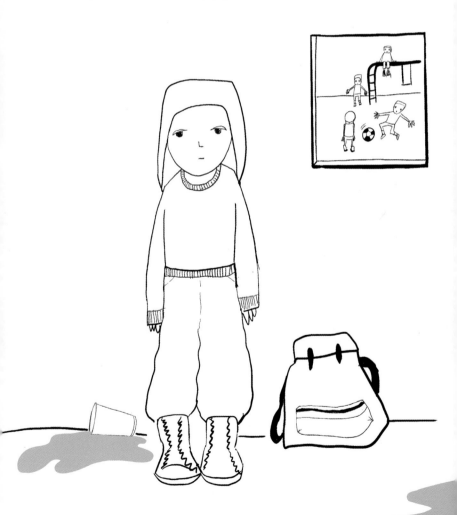

⬇ We might prefer to:

☐ walk slowly and carefully

☐ wear loose, baggy clothes

☐ avoid places where we might get bumped or crashed into

☐ hold things lightly (it might mean we drop them easily)

☐ avoid heights and climbing

☐ avoid lifting heavy things

☐ or something else!

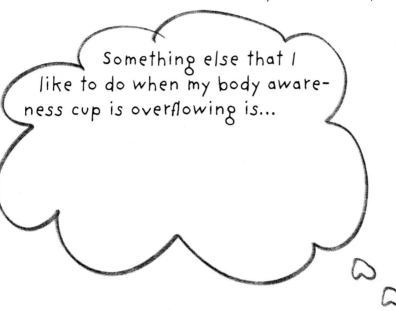

Something else that I like to do when my body awareness cup is overflowing is...

Sometimes our body awareness cup doesn't have enough information about where all of our different body parts are, and we need to do things to fill it back up.

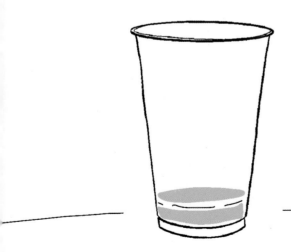

We might feel the need to...

- [ ] climb things

- [ ] chew our pens, pencils, nails or sleeves

- [ ] hold pens, scissors and other things really tightly

- [ ] walk on our tiptoes

- [ ] walk barefoot

- [ ] squeeze things

- [ ] swing our legs

- [ ] wear tighter clothes

- [ ] lean on people while talking to them

- [ ] sit with our legs crossed or under us

...to get back to the calm, happy, 'just right' feeling.

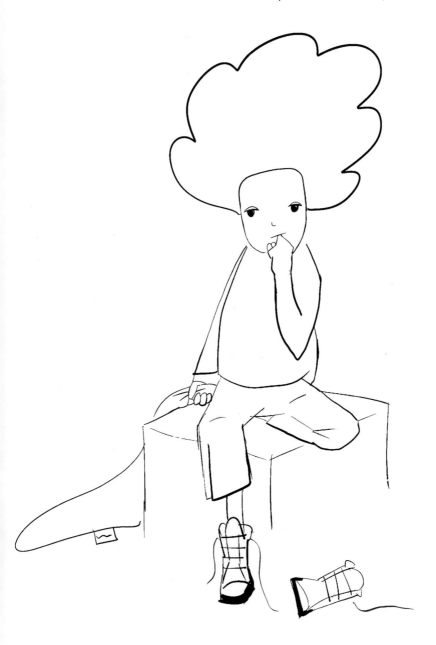

Do you do any of these things too? Tick them
off on the list.

Anything else? Write or draw it in the bubble.

# Inside Feelings Cup

And finally, the inside feelings sense! This is the one which helps us notice the feelings we get inside our body.

Are you feeling hungry? Tired? Angry? Sad? Do you need a wee? This is information that we get from inside our body including our inside organs, like our heart, lungs and stomach.

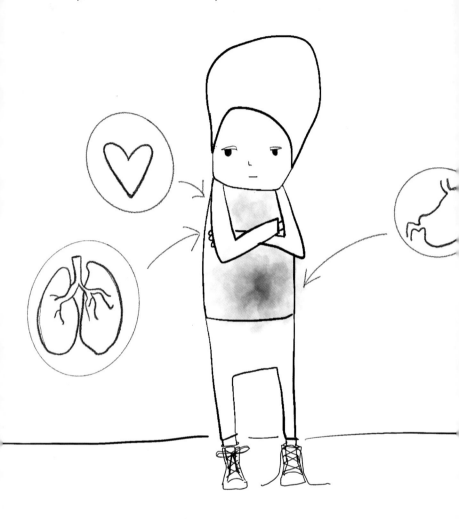

The long word for this sense is interoception (in-ter-o-sep-shun). But we'll call it our inside feelings sense to keep things easy.

It's how we know whether we are feeling...

* sick

* panicky

* cold

* in pain

* hot

* itchy

* like we need the toilet (and know how quickly we need to get there).

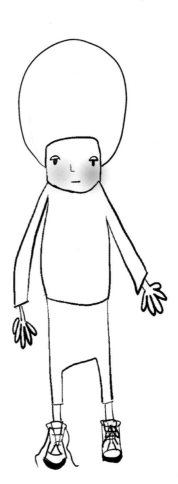

It tells us that we need to do **something** to get back to feeling 'just right'.

If we have too much information (or feelings we don't understand) in our inside feelings cup, it can be really, really confusing.

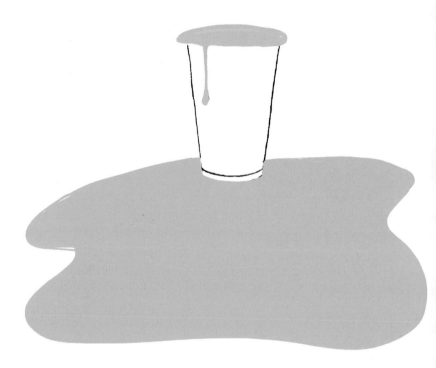

## We might... ⤓

- [ ] feel like we always need the toilet
- [ ] get easily hurt in small accidents
- [ ] forget to eat or drink
- [ ] feel too hot or too cold
- [ ] worry about our heartbeat
- [ ] feel itchy often
- [ ] panic when plasters need taking off
- [ ] feel like everything is just too much
- [ ] or something else.

Write yours here or tick any that have happened to you.

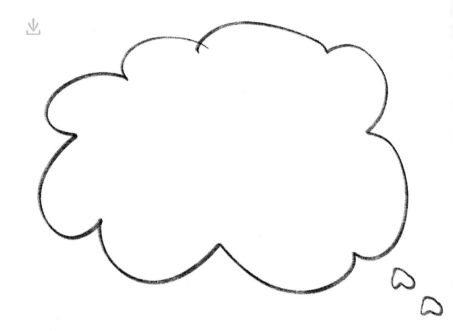

If our cup doesn't have enough information about things like needing the toilet, feeling pain or having an itch, it can be difficult to know what to do to get back to the calm, 'just right' feeling.

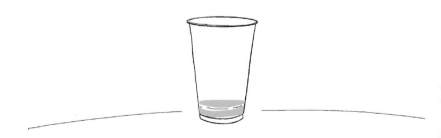

## We might...

- [ ] eat food, even when we aren't hungry

- [ ] drink more than we need

- [ ] not notice when we hurt ourselves

- [ ] not know we are in pain or not know **where** the pain is (but know it hurts)

- [ ] have difficulty working out what's making us itchy

- [ ] wear too many or too few clothes and overheat or freeze

- [ ] not make it to the toilet in time.

What about you? Tick any that you might have done.

What inside feelings are sometimes
'too much'?

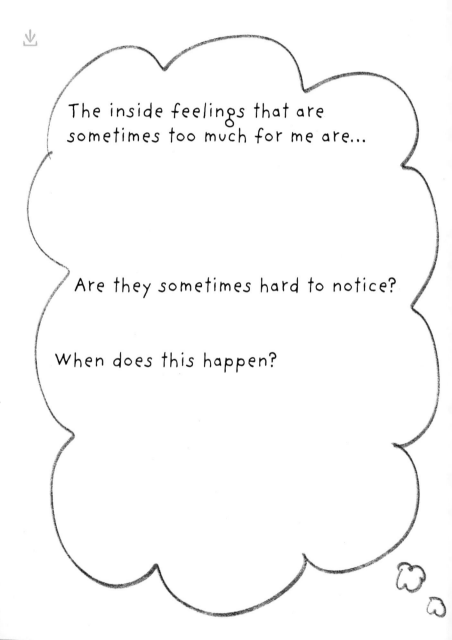

The inside feelings that are
sometimes too much for me are...

Are they sometimes hard to notice?

When does this happen?

Remember! At the end of the book and online, there are some ideas for what to do if your inside feelings are hard to notice and how to get back to feeling 'just right'.

And finally, there is one more, **very** important thing that interoception does.

Interoception also tells us about what **emotions**? we are feeling.

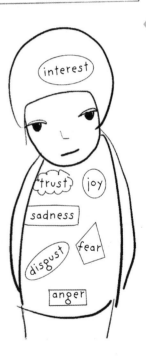

**Emotions**? are the labels we use to describe some of the inside feelings we get. Labels like happy, sad or angry.

87

These labels are useful because they can help us talk about how we feel.

Not everyone works the same way. We might have very different feelings (and labels) from the person next to us.

Even if we are seeing and hearing the same things.

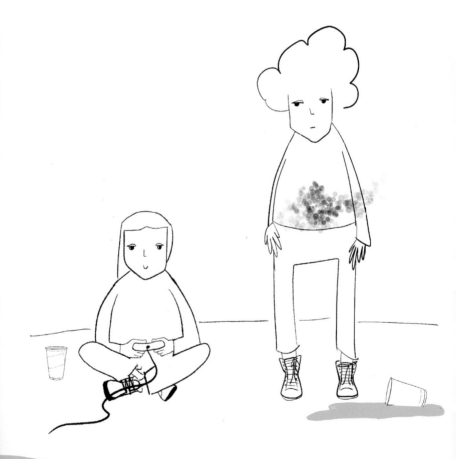

For one person, emotions might work like this:

* bubbly stomach + warm chest = surprise

* cold sinking feeling in stomach = fear

* heavy feeling on chest + tight throat = sadness

* hot hands + boiling feeling in stomach = anger

* fluttery feeling in chest and stomach = excitement

* sick feeling in stomach, throat and mouth = disgust.

For another person, they might work like this:

* fluttery chest = surprise

* fluttery chest = fear

* no inside feelings = sadness

* lots of different inside feelings = anger

* fluttery chest = excitement

* fluttery chest = disgust.

It can be very confusing!

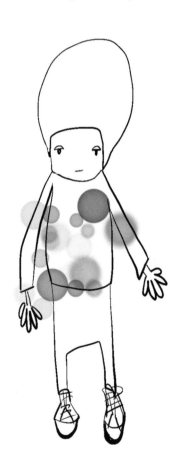

If we don't feel enough in our inside feelings cup, we might not get enough information. It can make it really hard to notice our emotions. We can end up feeling really uncertain.

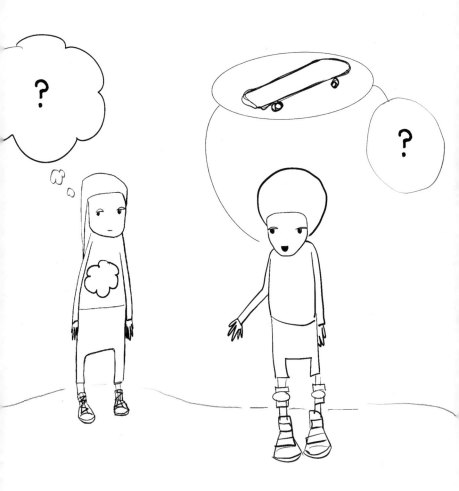

Knowing how we feel is really important for lots of reasons.

## Ten reasons why understanding our emotions is important

1. They can help us know if we like something.

2. They can help us know if we need to run away.

3. They can help us know if we like someone.

4. They can help us know if we love someone.

5. They can help us make choices.

6. They can help us explain if something is wrong.

7. They can help us know if we need to say no.

8. They can help us know if we need to fight back.

9. They can help us know if we want to message someone.

**And** it's also super important that...

**10.** ...they can help us understand how
other people might be feeling.

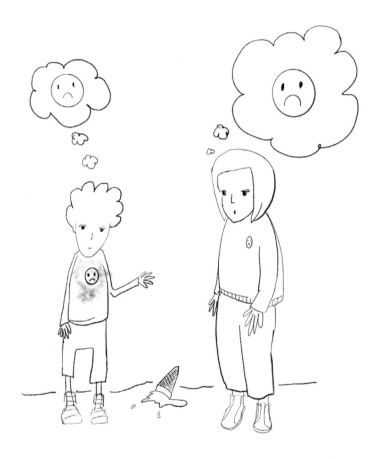

We may feel a little bit like they feel, and this
makes it easier for us to help them, or just to
connect, and understand how things are for
them that day.

Well done! You have learnt so much about our eight senses and our sense cups. In the next part of this book we are going to think a bit more about how different people's cups might look and work differently.

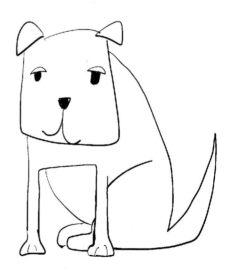

# PART 2

# SMALL cups,
# BIG cups,
# MEDIUM cups

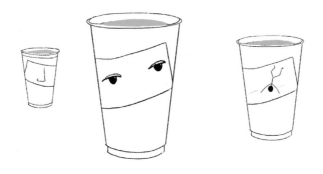

Everyone's cups are different sizes. And each of our eight cups might be different sizes. We might have a big sight cup but a small taste cup.

It's also important to know that sometimes our cups change size. They do this as we grow and develop. We might have a small taste cup when we are young and not like foods that are really full of flavour (like very spicy food). But as we get older our taste cup may get bigger, and we can then enjoy strong flavours.

The size of our cups can also change during the day, depending on where we are and if we are feeling calm or stressed – certain or uncertain. So this might mean we find some noises OK when we are relaxed but they are too much for us when we are stressed.

With people we know, in places we know, they might look like this:

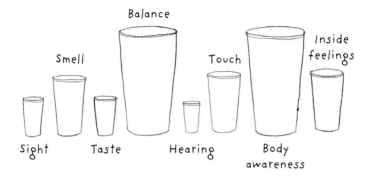

And in places we don't know, with people we don't know, they might look like this:

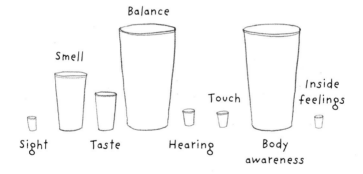

Some cups might shrink, so we get easily overwhelmed. Some cups might grow, so we need more information.

And that's OK. It's just our brain looking for the information it needs to keep us safe. It also makes it easier for us to feel overwhelmed.

Sometimes, when our cups are empty or spilling over, it can make us feel even more uncertain. This can make managing things like learning and friendships really difficult.

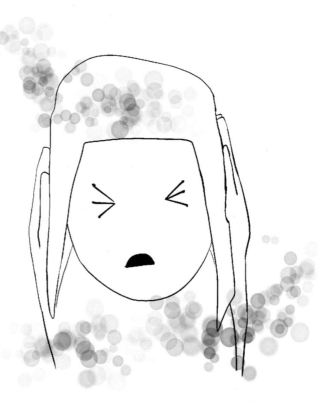

But, like we said in Part 1, by trying to learn more about our own cups and by noticing how our body is feeling, we can maybe start to feel a little less uncertain.

It can also remind us how fantastic our brains and bodies are and how they can give us information about what to do when we are feeling stressed or just 'not right'.

Learning about our sense cups, the way we understand and manage sensory information, helps us understand what can make us feel 'just right'. It also helps us understand why we might sometimes feel 'not right'. We can then make plans to use when we are feeling 'not right' that might help us out.

Now let's look at how your sense cups work.

# your unique sense cups

How does **your** unique set of sense cups work?

Did you fill in some of the pages in Part 1?
Think about what you did while you did this.
Did you sit on your heels? Did you chew your
pen? Did you move around?

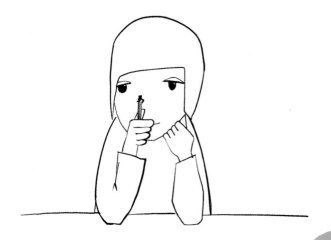

So, what next?

The good news is that you've already taken the first step.

Knowing more about how our bodies and brains work can help us understand what's going on when we feel fidgety, overwhelmed or 'not right'.

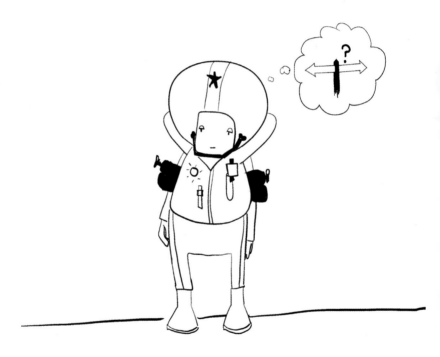

It's our body's way of trying to keep us safe and work out what we should do next to get back to the 'just right' feeling.

Read on if you would like some ideas on what to do when your cups are too full (overflowing) or too empty.

## Me and my cups

How much you like the next bit of this book depends on you and how much you like experiments.

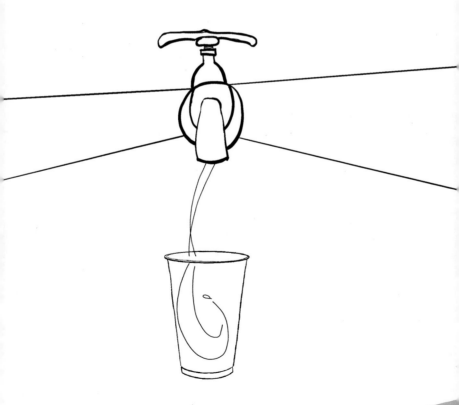

# Filling and Emptying your Cups

These next few pages are here to give you some ideas about things you can do to fill or empty your cups to get back to feeling 'just right'. There are some more ideas online, too.

Feeling 'not quite right'? Try these three things.

1.  **Breathe slowly and notice what's going on in all the different parts of your body. See if you can notice where the 'not right' feeling is strongest.**

    It can feel a bit weird when you first do this.

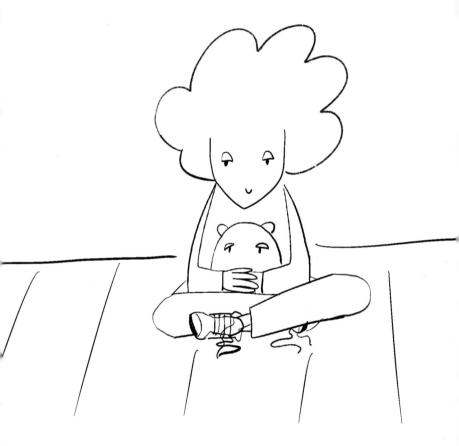

Don't worry. It gets easier with practice.

**2. See if you can notice more about those feelings.**

Are they big or small?

Are they moving or still?

Are they hot or cold?

What colour would they be?

Could you draw them on a piece of paper?
Do it!

Could you draw them on an outline of your body? You could have a go here on the outline below. (This is based on Jamie's body – he is tall and has no hair!)

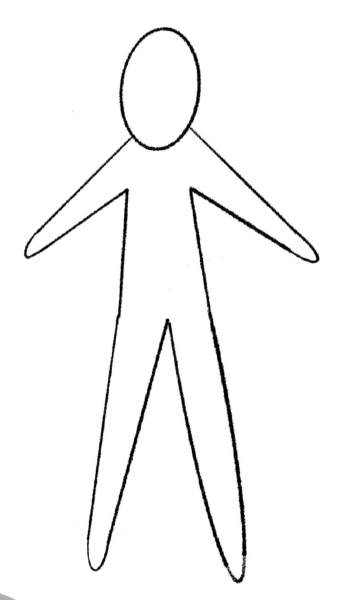

**3. Have a go at some of the activities on the next few pages and have a look online.**

If something helps you get back to feeling 'just right', write it down at the end of this book and tell someone about it, so they can remind you next time.

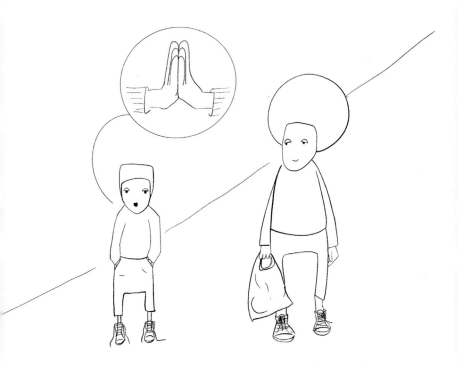

Because there will be a next time. Listening to these messages from your body is how you work out what it needs. And that's a good thing.

Feeling fidgety in a lesson?

You may have too much or too little in some of your cups.

Try keeping some small objects in your pocket, school bag or pencil case.

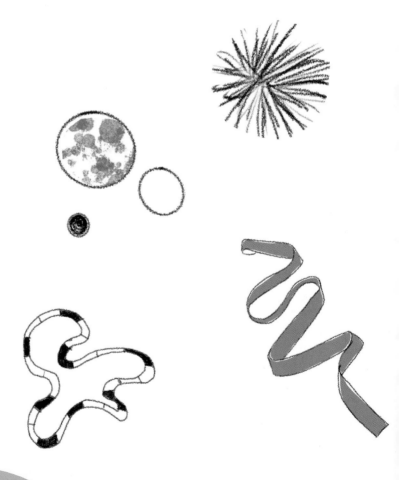

And here's the really important bit: you might want to talk to your teacher if you're going to use these things in lessons as our fidgeting can make other people's cups overflow.

(Squeeze balls, twist and lock blocks, tangles, rubber bands, ribbons, bits of material and Velcro dots are good, quiet fidgets.)

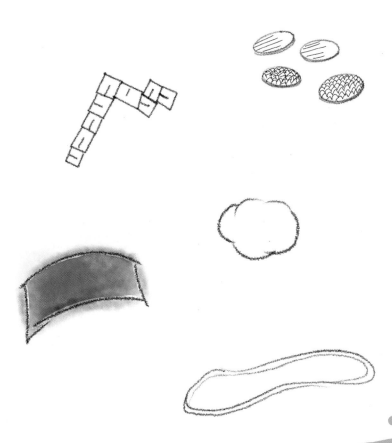

Feeling low energy?

Ask your teacher
if you can stand
(at the side or the
back of the room)
for some of the lesson.
Explain that you are
experimenting with
what helps you concentrate
and show them this book.

standing desk

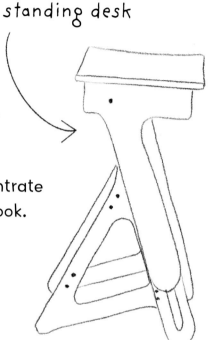

elastic

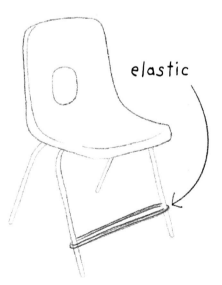

Buy a 1.5 metre
length of elastic
and tie it so it fits
across the front
legs of a chair.
Press or bounce
your feet against
it as you work.

Make a poster or digital presentation to persuade your school to buy some balance ball chairs or standing desks. You could even do some fundraising to buy them.

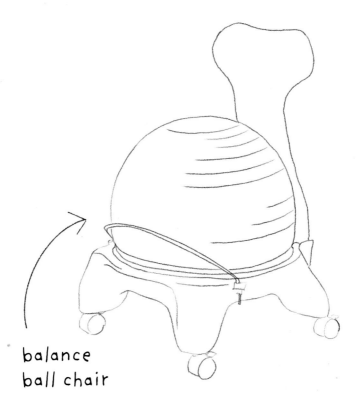

balance
ball chair

Feeling overwhelmed?

Try some secret chair yoga (no one will know):

1. Press your feet firmly into the floor.

2. Let your breath flow. Imagine the air is doing all the work, moving gently in and out of your lungs.

3. Try some of these gentle stretches.

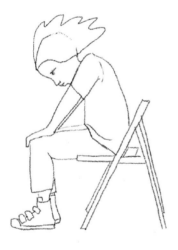

Push

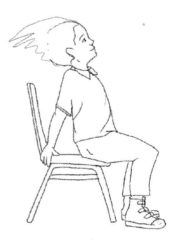

Twist

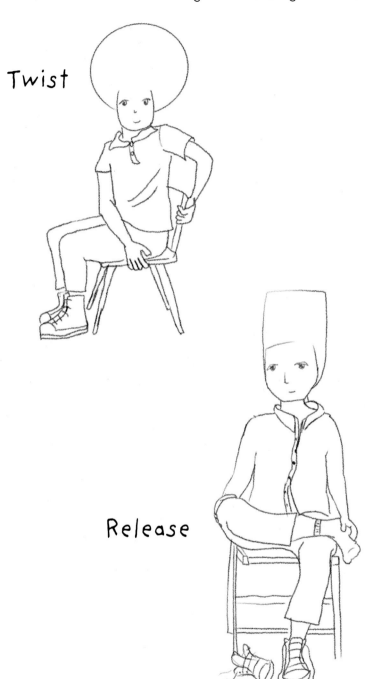

Release

Hopefully you now know a bit more about yourself and your sense cups. And that your cups will change size depending on where you are and what you are doing.

See if you can draw your cups in each of these situations. Go back to the start of Part 2 to see how different cups can be different sizes, like when we are in a place we know or a place we don't know.

Usually my cups are:

⬇

Touch  Taste  Smell  Sight  Hearing  Balance  Proprioception  Interoception

When I am stressed, my cups are...

Touch   Taste   Smell   Sight   Hearing   Balance   Proprioception   Interoception

Things I can do that help me get back
to feeling 'just right'...

_____

_____

_____

_____

_____

_____

_____

_____

_____

_____

_____

Well done! You've made it to the end of the book. Hopefully you've learned a few things along the way. Maybe you discovered some senses you didn't know you had?

Some of you might have found it tricky thinking about your sense cups. That's OK. By making it this far you are off to a great start!

We are always learning more about our own unique brains and bodies, even as grown-ups! The important thing is that we stay curious and keep noticing and learning. Just like you have done in keeping going to the end of this book.

The more we learn about ourselves, our uniquely brilliant way of being and how we are sensing the world and reacting to it, the more chance we have of noticing and managing when we are feeling 'not right' or confused. And when we notice that we are not feeling quite right and which of our senses needs more or less input, that's a big step towards getting ourselves back to feeling 'just right' again.

If you'd like some more ideas for what to do to get back to feeling 'just right', have a look online.

Happy experimenting!

---

'My Senses Are Like Cups' is one of a range of materials based on the 3S framework for understanding uncertainty and anxiety. The framework can be used to 'unpick' causes of stress and guides parents and practitioners to understand experiences as a combination of three types of uncertainty: structure, sensory (as described in this book) and social before designing support.

Visit www.specialnetworks.co.uk for more information.

# THE ANXIETY WORKBOOK

for Supporting Teens Who Learn Differently

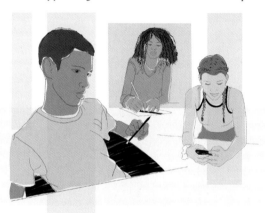

A Framework and Activities to Build Structural,
Sensory and Social Certainty

BY CLARE WARD AND JAMIE GALPIN • FOREWORDS BY SARAH WILD AND PROFESSOR LIZ PELLICANO
ILLUSTRATED BY CLARE WARD WITH ORLA LATHAM

**The Anxiety Workbook for Supporting
Teens Who Learn Differently**

A Framework and Activities to Build
Structural, Sensory and Social Certainty

Clare Ward and Jamie Galpin

Illustrated by Clare Ward

Foreword by Kelly Mahler

ISBN 978 1 78775 396 9

eISBN 978 1 78775 397 6

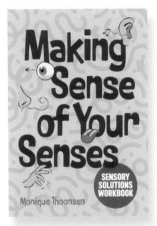

**Making Sense of Your Senses**
Sensory Solutions Workbook
Monique Thoonsen
Illustrated by Ruud Bijman
ISBN 978 1 83997 802 9
eISBN 978 1 83997 811 1

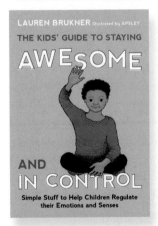

**The Kids' Guide to Staying Awesome and In Control**
Simple Stuff to Help Children Regulate their Emotions and Senses
Lauren Brukner
Illustrated by Apsley
ISBN 978 1 84905 997 8
eISBN 978 0 85700 962 3

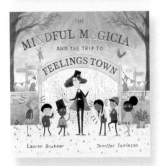

**The Mindful Magician and the Trip to Feelings Town**
Tips and Tricks to Help the Youngest Readers Regulate their Emotions and Senses
Lauren Brukner
Illustrated by Jennifer Jamieson
ISBN 978 1 83997 138 9
eISBN 978 1 83997 139 6